THE
BodyBook

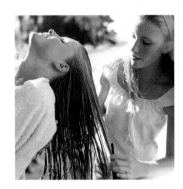

Anne Akers Johnson

KLUTZ

KLUTZ® is a kids' company staffed entirely by real human beings. We began our corporate life in 1977 in an office we shared with a Chevrolet Impala. Today we've outgrown our founding garage, but Palo Alto, California, remains Klutz galactic headquarters. For those of you who collect corporate mission statements, here's ours:

CREATE WONDERFUL THINGS · BE GOOD · HAVE FUN

Write Us

We would love to hear your comments regarding this or any of our books. We have many!

KLUTZ®

455 Portage Avenue
Palo Alto, CA 94306
Visit Us: ☞ **KLUTZ**.com

Printed in Singapore.

Nail file and buffer made in Korea;
all other spa box contents made in Taiwan.

The "book and box" format is a registered trademark of Klutz, Inc.

Additional Copies and More Supplies:
For the location of your nearest Klutz retailer, call (650) 857-0888. Should they be tragically out of stock, additional copies of this book, replacement spa boxes and the entire library of 100% Klutz certified books are available in our mail order catalog. See the last page for details.

Klutz is a Nelvana company

contents

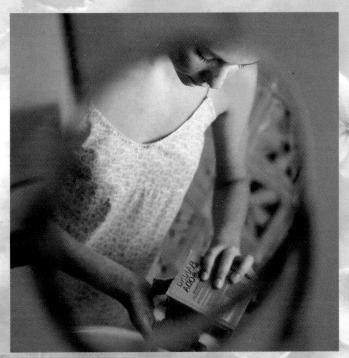

It will come as no surprise to you that natural body care starts on the inside. Treat your body right and you've done most of the work necessary for beautiful skin, hair and nails. The basics are simple:

Water

Try to drink 6–8 glasses of water a day (8 ounces each). Caffeinated drinks and milk don't count. Herbal teas and fruit juices do.

Food

Eat a balanced diet to ensure your body gets all the nutrients it needs. Veggies and fruit are great. Limit fried foods and sweets. But you already knew that.

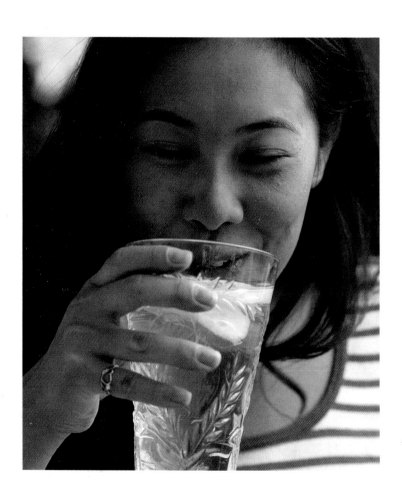

INTROD

Sleep

Most people need a full 8 hours of sleep every day to feel well and rested. If you feel good, you look good. It's a fact.

Exercise

Aside from keeping your body fit and strong, exercise helps cleanse your system of toxins. Experts recommend you do some kind of aerobic exercise 3–4 times a week for at least 20 minutes. Try to find an activity you enjoy so this isn't a chore.

Sun

This is a big one. How well you protect your skin in the first 20 years of your life impacts the health (and look) of your skin for the rest of your life. Always wear sun screen (at least spf 15) when you're going to be out in the sun for a prolonged period. Wear hats. Get over the idea that you need a tan to look good. It's just not good for your skin.

The all-important patch test

While all the ingredients used in this book are natural, it's a good idea to do a patch test before you slather a new concoction on your face or body. Simply apply a small amount of the recipe to the inside of your forearm. Keep the area small, about one inch square. Cover it with an adhesive strip and leave it on for 24 hours. If your skin burns, itches or turns red, it means you're reacting to one of the ingredients and should not use it on your body. Wash the recipe off with warm, soapy water. If you have especially sensitive skin check with your dermatologist before trying the recipes in this book.

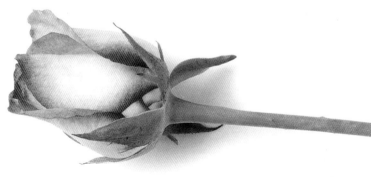

UCTION

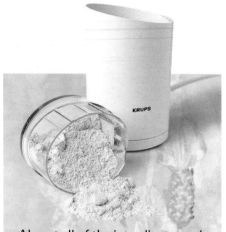

Almost all of the ingredients used in this book can be picked up at your local grocery store, natural food store or pharmacy.

Many recipes call for grinding beans or oatmeal into a flour. A blender or food processor will work fine for this, though they're both a little large for the quantities you'll be working with. Consider buying a small coffee bean grinder (about $15) that you can dedicate to your natural recipes. Just be sure no one uses it to grind their coffee, or everything you make will smell like coffee beans.

This book comes with a complete home spa kit. As you read through the book you'll find out just how to use each item in the kit. This is everything you get:

- facial brush: use to clean your face

- headband: holds your hair back off your face

- nail brush: use to clean your nails

- nail file: shapes your nails

- buffer: a natural alternative to nail polish

- pumice stone: smooths rough spots on your feet

- shower cap: covers your hair during hair masks

- muslin bag: holds your bath infusions

- essential oil: scents your spa recipes

A note about essential oil

Your spa kit comes with three kinds of essential oil: lavender, mint and tangerine. Though many of the recipes in this book call for a specific scent, feel free to substitute one for the other, or even to blend the oils to make your own scent.

You can usually buy essential oil from natural food stores or bath shops. They're often mixed with a different, unscented oil to dilute them a bit. This isn't a bad thing. Some essential oils can be irritating to your skin if they're pure. Always read the label before using a new essential oil. Be sure to do a patch test whenever you use a new scent. Fiddle around with how much oil you add to your concoctions. Each new scent and each brand will vary in strength so you may need to add a little more or a little less than called for. Your best plan when starting out with a new essential oil is to add a drop at a time until you've got the scent just right.

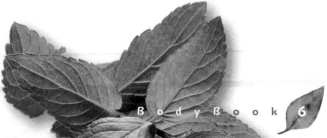

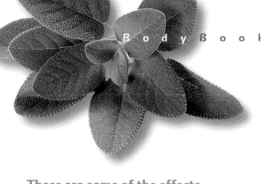

These are some of the effects essential oil can have:

- Lavender: leaves you feeling calmed and relaxed. Good just before you go to bed.

- Lemon: uplifting and clarifying. Also a good astringent.

- Peppermint: stimulating, leaves your skin feeling fresh and your mind clear.

- Rose: uplifting and soothing, also a little expensive.

- Tangerine: a soothing scent that helps you feel relaxed.

- Rosemary: an energizing astringent that can help prevent dandruff.

Because essential oils can damage countertops and other household surfaces, it's a good idea to spread newspaper over your work area before you get started.

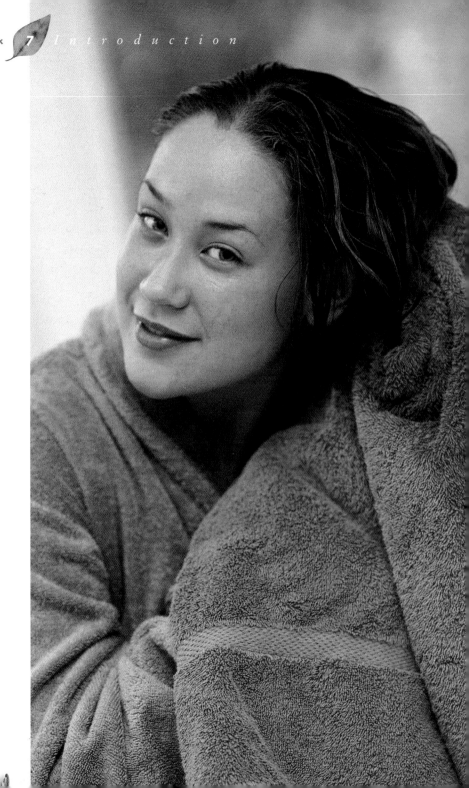

F

SCRUBS & STEAMS & MASKS & EYE

ACE

SOOTHERS & TONERS & THE COMPLETE FACIAL

scrubs

It's important to establish a daily routine for keeping your skin clean and toned. The scrubs in this section are a great way to start. It's usually enough to wash your face with a cleanser or scrub once a day, just before you go to bed. This removes any impurities that have accumulated during the day, as well as makeup you may have applied. In the morning it's enough to simply rinse your face in warm water and pat it dry with a clean dry towel. Over-cleansing can throw your skin off balance, causing it to produce more oil and leading to breakouts.

Of course, if a dermatologist has prescribed a routine specific to your skin, check with her before doing anything different.

Applying a scrub

· All of these recipes make enough for one scrub and are applied in pretty much the same way. Use your fingers or the facial brush that comes with this book.

· First splash your face with warm water. If you're using the brush, get it wet as well.

· Scoop the scrub onto your brush or fingers and work it all over your face using gentle circular motions. Never press hard or tug on your skin. Avoid your eye area. If you get something in your eyes, rinse them immediately with water.

· Rinse your face with warm (never hot) water, then pat it dry with a clean, soft towel.

· If you used your facial brush, rinse it clean under running water. Store it where it will dry between uses. Don't put the cap on unless the brush is dry. Discard any unused scrub.

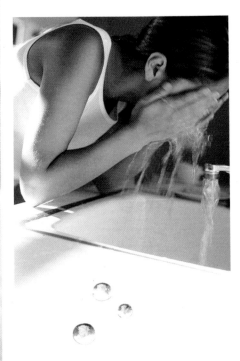

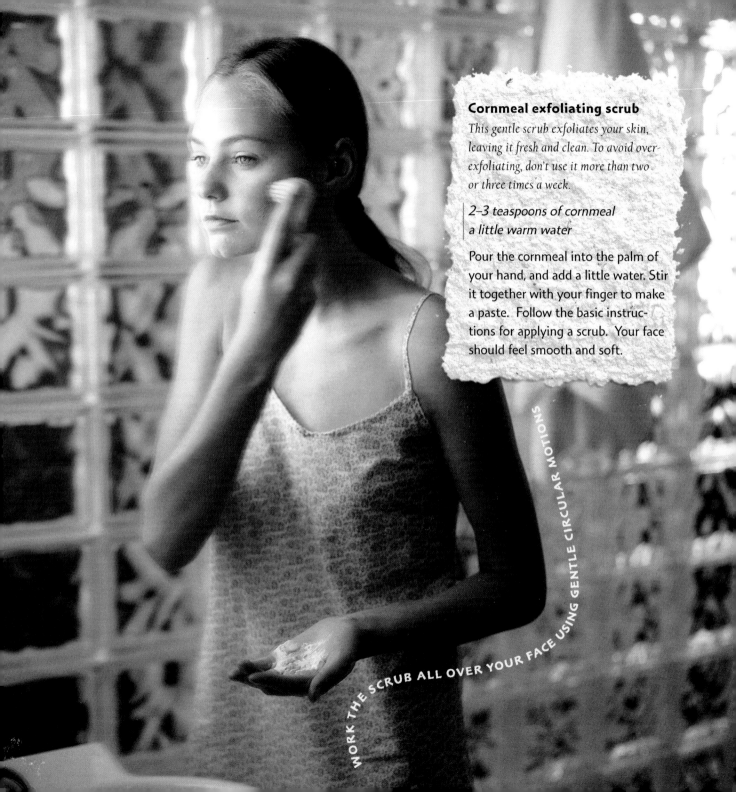

Cornmeal exfoliating scrub

This gentle scrub exfoliates your skin, leaving it fresh and clean. To avoid over-exfoliating, don't use it more than two or three times a week.

2–3 teaspoons of cornmeal
a little warm water

Pour the cornmeal into the palm of your hand, and add a little water. Stir it together with your finger to make a paste. Follow the basic instructions for applying a scrub. Your face should feel smooth and soft.

WORK THE SCRUB ALL OVER YOUR FACE USING GENTLE CIRCULAR MOTIONS

Extra gentle, everyday polishing scrub

This gentle scrub works well on all skin types and, as the name suggests, it's gentle enough to use every day. It will leave your face feeling soft and clean.

2–3 tsp of baking soda
a little warm water

Pour the baking soda into the palm of your hand. Mix in enough water to make a paste, then apply with your fingers or facial brush as always.

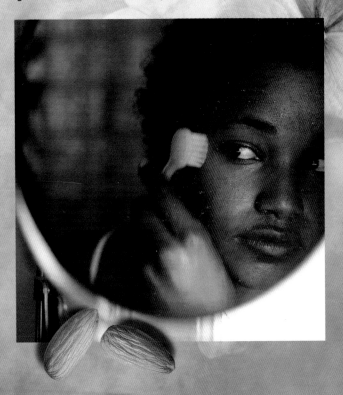

Strawberry almond scrub

Strawberries have natural astringent properties that tighten your pores, and leave your face feeling toned and fresh. Try grinding a quarter-cup of almonds at once, and store them in a jar in the refrigerator so you always have some around.

2 tsp baking soda
1 tsp ground almonds
1 ripe strawberry (If fresh strawberries aren't available, it's OK to use thawed, frozen berries.)

Mix the almonds and baking soda together in a small dish.

Slice a single strawberry into the bowl and mash it all together with a fork (or your fingers) to make a smooth paste.

Apply to your face using your facial brush or your fingertips as directed in the basic scrub instructions.

Almond rose scrub

The almonds and rosewater in this recipe combine to smooth and hydrate your skin. If you don't have rosewater, plain water works fine. But really, use rosewater. Check page 29 for information on where you can find it.

1 Tbsp ground almonds
1 tsp rosewater or water

Mix the almonds and water to a paste, then apply to your face using your facial brush or your fingertips.

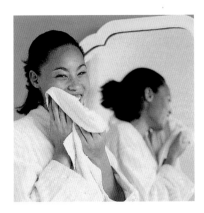

Milk and honey scrub

The almonds cleanse and exfoliate your skin, while the milk and honey moisturize it. Use nonfat milk if your skin tends to be oily, whole milk or even cream if your skin is dry.

1 Tbsp ground almonds
1 tsp honey
1 tsp milk or cream

Mix all the ingredients together in a small dish, then apply to your face as usual.

Azuki bean scrub

This is a good scrub for normal to oily skin. It's an excellent exfoliant and helps to clear blackheads. You'll need a blender, food processor or a clean coffee grinder to make it. If you can't find azuki beans at your usual grocery store, check at a natural foods store. This recipe makes enough for about six scrubs.

½ cup dried azuki beans

Pour the dry beans into a blender, food processor or, even better, a clean coffee grinder. Grind the beans to the consistency of a coarse flour (like cornmeal). Be sure to put the cover on tightly first, or you'll be pelted by flying beans. Store in a dry jar or plastic bag until ready to use.

TO USE: Pour 2–3 teaspoons of ground beans into the palm of your hand. Add a little water and stir with your finger to make a paste. Scoop up with your fingers or a damp facial brush and apply as usual.

Oatmeal scrub

Oats have been used for years to tone and soften skin. The lemon works as an astringent, while the yogurt soothes and lightly moisturizes. Grind a larger batch of oatmeal and keep it around so you can mix this scrub up easily. Always use regular oats, not the instant kind.

1 Tbsp ground oatmeal
1 tsp lemon juice
2 tsp yogurt

Combine the ingredients in a small bowl, then apply as always.

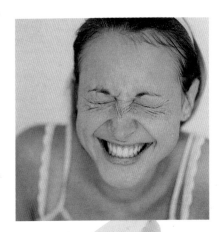

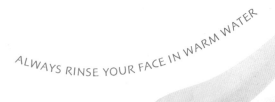

ALWAYS RINSE YOUR FACE IN WARM WATER

steams

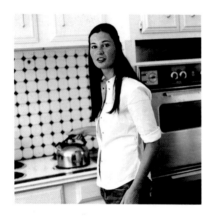

Steams are a soothing and aromatic way to deep clean your skin. The gentle heat opens and cleanses your pores while hydrating your skin. They also double as aromatherapy treatments. Try adding a facial steam to your once-a-week routine. If your face is broken out at the moment, save this treatment for another day. The heat stimulates your skin, and can aggravate already-irritated skin.

The basic facial steam

- Start by washing your face with your regular cleanser, or with one of the scrubs in this book.

- Choose a steam recipe and assemble as directed. Pour it into a medium-sized bowl. The steam should be warm enough that you can feel the heat rise off of it. Anything over 140°F is too hot and could burn you.

- Pull your hair back off your face and lean over the bowl. Drape a towel over your head and the bowl to catch the steam. Relax and enjoy your steam for about 10 minutes.

- After the steam, splash your face with cool water, then pat it dry. Follow with one of the toners on page 26–29 if you'd like.

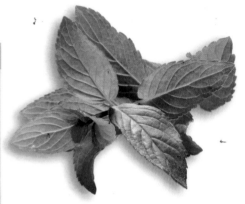

Minty steam

This is a refreshing, energizing steam. It's an especially good choice if you're feeling under the weather and could use a boost.

4 cups warm tap water
4 mint tea bags (use herbal tea only) or a handful of fresh mint, slightly crushed

Bring two cups of water to a boil then remove from heat.

Add the mint and let it steep for a minute before adding the remaining two cups of warm tap water.

Follow the basic steam directions.

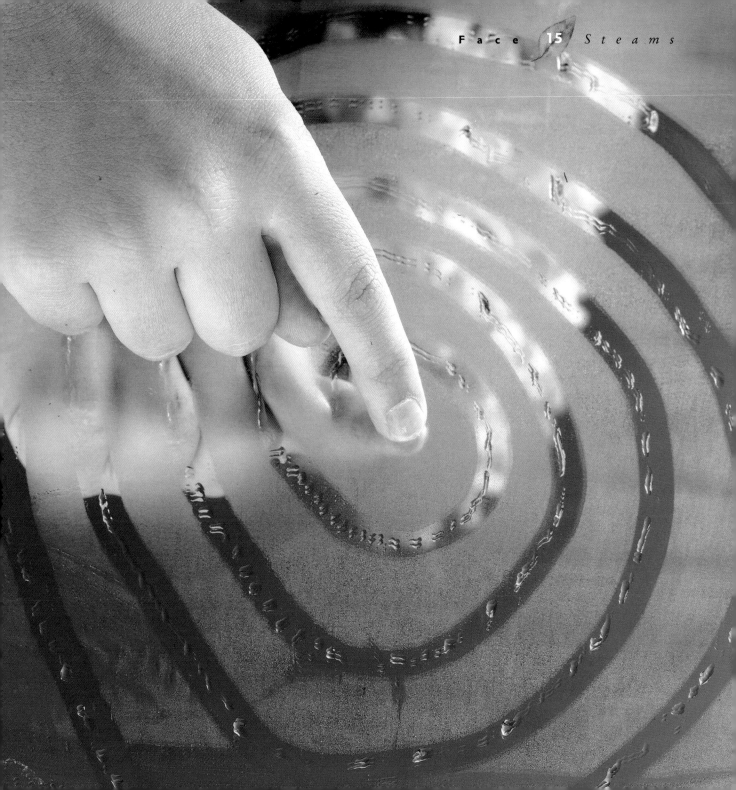

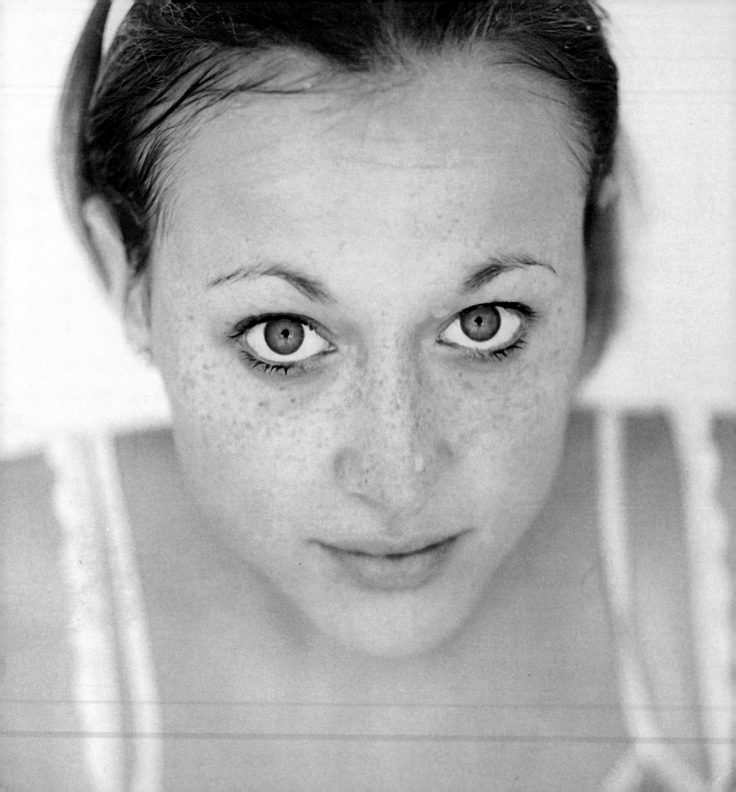

Clarifying citrus steam

This clarifying steam will leave your skin feeling fresh and thoroughly clean.

4 cups warm tap water
1 lemon, cut into ¼-inch slices
2 drops tangerine essential oil

Bring two cups of water to a boil then remove from heat.

Add the lemon slices to the water, being careful not to splash, and let it steep for a minute before adding the essential oil and the remaining two cups of warm tap water.

Follow the basic steam directions.

Herbal steam

Choose rosemary, sage, or a mix of the two for this aromatic, toning steam. Both herbs have astringent and antiseptic qualities that will leave your skin feeling clean and hydrated.

4 cups warm tap water
4 Tbsp dried rosemary and/or sage
 or
a handful of fresh rosemary and/or
 sage

Bring two cups of water to a boil then remove from heat.

Add the herbs and let them steep for a minute before adding the remaining two cups of warm tap water.

Follow the basic steam directions.

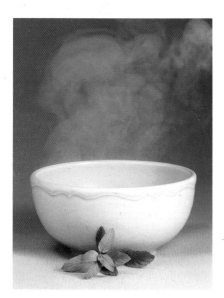

Lavender steam

Lavender is known for the soothing and toning effects it can have on your skin. Its scent will leave you feeling rested.

4 cups warm tap water
8–10 drops lavender essential oil

Bring two cups of water to a boil then remove from heat.

Add the essential oil and the remaining two cups of water.

Follow the directions for a steam on page 14.

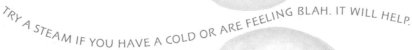

TRY A STEAM IF YOU HAVE A COLD OR ARE FEELING BLAH. IT WILL HELP.

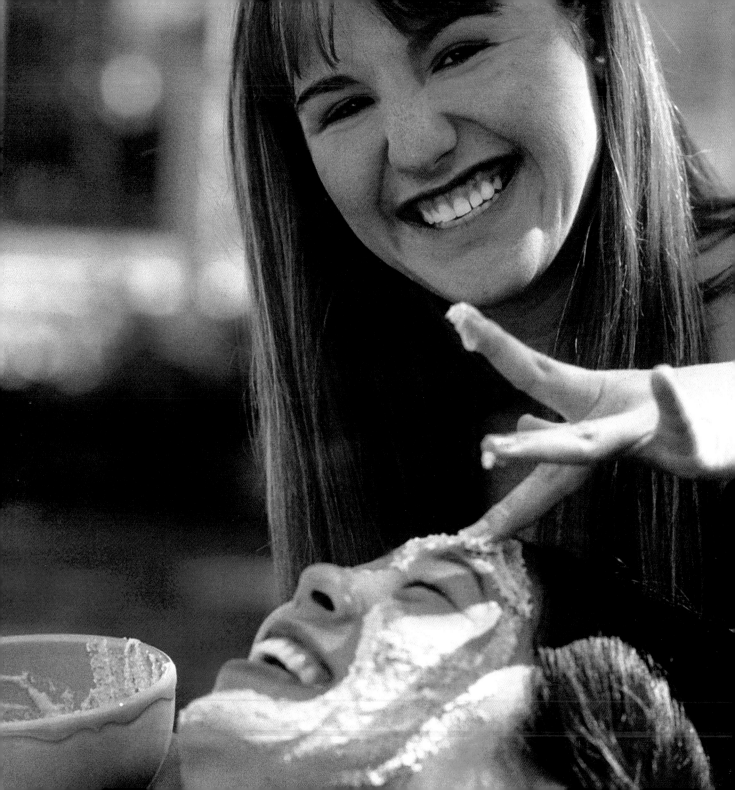

masks

Masks are intensive treatments and should be limited to your once-a-week routine. Choose one that is well suited to your skin.

Basic facial mask

- Before applying a mask, find a place where you can lie back without being disturbed. Spread a towel out where you will rest your head in case your mask drips.

- Choose and prepare a recipe.

- Pull your hair back off your face. The headband that came with this book is perfect for this. Pull long hair back into a ponytail.

- Wash your face so it's nice and clean.

- Run a washcloth under warm water, squeeze it out and hold it over your face for a few seconds to dampen your face. If you've just had a steam, skip this step.

- Apply the mask all over your face and neck (if you like), avoiding your eye area. Lie back and let the mask work for 10–15 minutes. If it starts to feel itchy or uncomfortable, less time is OK.

- If your mask is particularly chunky (like oatmeal) use your washcloth to gently wipe it off your face, shaking the bits of mask into the trash (this is the trick to avoiding clogged drains). Once it's mostly off, rinse your face in warm water.

- Discard any leftover mask.

Simple oatmeal mask

This mask works well on all skin types. If your skin is dry, use whole milk or cream, otherwise stick to low fat or nonfat milk. Oatmeal will leave your skin feeling soft and toned.

3 Tbsp regular, uncooked oatmeal, ground to a fine flour
2 Tbsp milk or cream

Combine all the ingredients in a small bowl. Follow the basic instructions for applying a mask.

Oatmeal honey mask

This is another very simple mask that takes advantage of oatmeal's cleansing and softening qualities. The honey lightly hydrates your skin. This mask helps to clear blackheads.

3 Tbsp regular, uncooked oatmeal
2 Tbsp honey

Combine the two ingredients in a bowl, then apply to your face as always. Rinse off after 10 minutes.

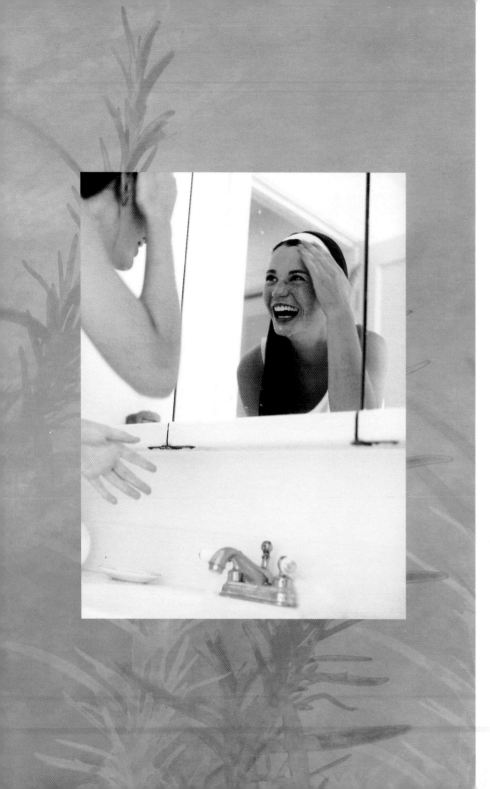

Honey souffle mask

The eggs and honey in this recipe work to tighten your pores and gently hydrate your skin. Always keep raw egg away from broken skin.

1 egg white
1 tsp honey
2 drops of lavender essential oil
  (optional but nice)

In a small bowl, beat the egg white until it is frothy and forms peaks. Gently fold in the honey and essential oil if you're using it.

Apply the mask to your face as always and let sit for 10 minutes before thoroughly rinsing your face.

Banana honey mask

This mask is good for all skin types and will leave your face soft and lightly mois- turized.

½ ripe banana
1 Tbsp honey

Mash the ingredients together completely.

Apply to your face as always and let it work for 10–15 minutes. Rinse your face with warm water.

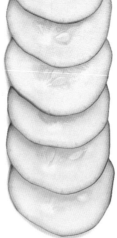

Apple mask

Good for all skin types. The ingredients in this mask work to tone and soften your skin.

½ *apple, grated into a bowl*
2 *tsp honey*
1 *Tbsp uncooked, regular oatmeal*

Grind the oatmeal into a flour in a clean coffee grinder or food processor if you have one. Unground oatmeal is OK too, it just makes the mask a little messier.

Combine all the ingredients.

Lie back and gently press small handfuls of the mask onto your face. Rub it along the sides of your face, then let it sit for 10–15 minutes before removing and rinsing.

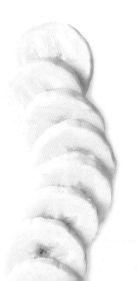

Extra gentle yogurt mask

This mask is a good choice if you have sensitive skin. The yogurt and cucumber combine to leave your skin feeling soft and gently toned. Choose whole milk yogurt if your skin is dry, otherwise nonfat or low fat will work best for you.

¼ *cup yogurt*
¼ *cucumber, peeled*

Place the yogurt and cucumber in a blender or food processor and puree until smooth. Pour it into a bowl and use a cotton pad to pat the mask all over your face. It will be a little runny.

Let the mask work for about 10 minutes before rinsing off.

Avo moisturizing mask

Try this mask if you have normal to dry skin. The avocado moisturizes, while the lemon acts as a balancing astringent.

½ *ripe avocado*
1 *lemon wedge (about ¼ of a whole lemon)*

Remove the flesh of the avocado from the skin and place it in a bowl. Squeeze the lemon over avocado to get about 1 tsp of juice out of it.

Mash the two ingredients together until the avocado is smooth or you're tired of mashing.

Apply to your face as always, letting the mask work for 10–15 minutes.

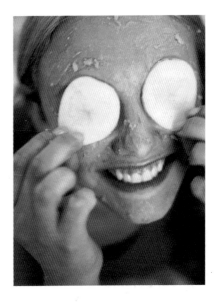

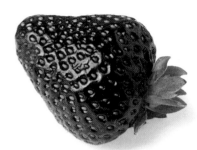
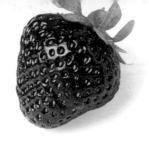

Strawberry mask

Strawberries have astringent qualities which tighten and tone your skin.

3–4 ripe strawberries (It's OK to thaw frozen strawberries if fresh aren't available.)

Mash the strawberries in a small bowl. Apply to your face as directed in the basic mask instructions and and leave on for 10–15 minutes before rinsing off.

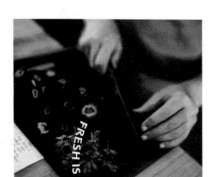

Tropical fruit masks

Both pineapple and papaya contain an enzyme that breaks down dead skin cells so they can be washed away, leaving your skin feeling fresh and clarified. Pineapple is more potent, papaya more gentle.

If you don't want to tackle a whole pineapple for this simple mask, check the produce section of your grocery store for already-cut pineapple. If you can't find it there, try the salad bar.

Papaya is trickier. If you can't find it fresh look for frozen fruit. Once you have your fresh pineapple or papaya, consider freezing pre-cut chunks, which you can thaw and use when fresh isn't available.

1 bite-sized chunk pineapple or papaya

Make sure your face is rinsed clean of makeup.

Rub the fruit all over your face to coat your skin with its juice. As always avoid your eye area.

Lie back and let the mask work. Don't be surprised if your skin tingles as the fruit enzymes go to work. If it becomes itchy or uncomfortable, rinse your face in warm water right away, otherwise leave it on for 10 minutes before rinsing. Your face might be a little pink after this treatment, but it will soon return to normal (but cleaner).

FRESH IS ALWAYS BEST, BUT IT'S OK TO SUBSTITUTE CANNED OR FROZEN FRUIT IF YOU HAVE TO

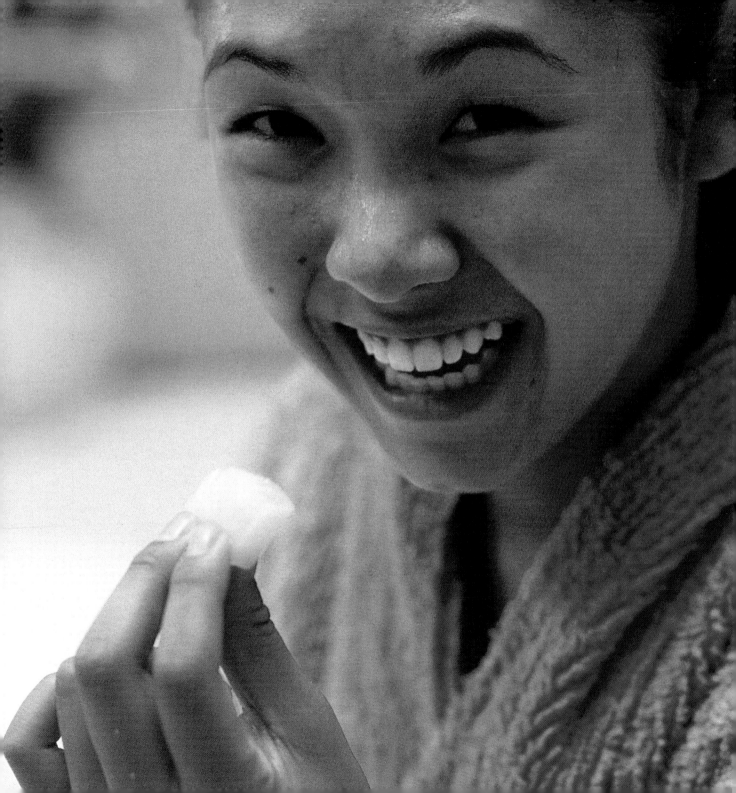

While you're lying back enjoying your mask, try placing an eye soother over your eyes. These soothers not only feel good, they help reduce puffiness under your eyes.

soothers

Using an eye soother

- Run a clean washcloth under cold water, put it in a bowl and chill in the refrigerator for 20 minutes. If you can't wait, simply dunk the washcloth in a bowl of ice water.

- Squeeze the towel out then fold it in half lengthwise two times to make a long narrow band.

- When you're ready, lie back and place the soother over your closed eyes, then drape the folded-up towel over them.

- Leave the soother on for 5–10 minutes. If the soother is uncomfortable, remove it at immediately and rinse your eyes with cool water. Discontinue use.

- Discard eye soother after use.

Black tea soother

Black tea contains tannin, which reduces the puffiness around your eyes. Cheaper teas tend to have a higher tannin level, so don't waste your money on the fancy stuff.

2 black tea bags

Run the tea bags under cool water to completely moisten the tea.

Being careful of the staples in the bags (if there are any) place the damp tea bags over your closed eyes. Cover with a cool washcloth and relax for 5–10 minutes.

Potato soother

If you think of it, chill the potato in the refrigerator for about an hour before using.

2 thin slices raw potato

Place one slice of potato over each eye, then cover with a cool washcloth for 5–10 minutes.

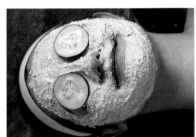

Cucumber soother

This classic treatment will leave you feeling refreshed.

thin cucumber slices (It's nice if the cucumber is thin enough to bend a little.)

Place the cucumbers over your closed eyes, then cover with a cool washcloth for 5–10 minutes.

This lightly flavored water makes it easy to drink your 8 glasses a day. Mix up a big batch and have it on hand to sip while you're getting a natural spa treatment.

1 cucumber
½ lemon
water

Peel the cucumber (important) and slice it into a big pitcher.

Slice the lemon half into rounds and add them to the pitcher as well.

Fill the pitcher with water and chill in the refrigerator for at least an hour.

After pouring yourself a glass of spa water, you can refill the pitcher to make more. It's best to toss the water and make a new batch from scratch after 24 hours.

This recipe is even better if you add a sliced apple or pear to the cucumbers and lemon.

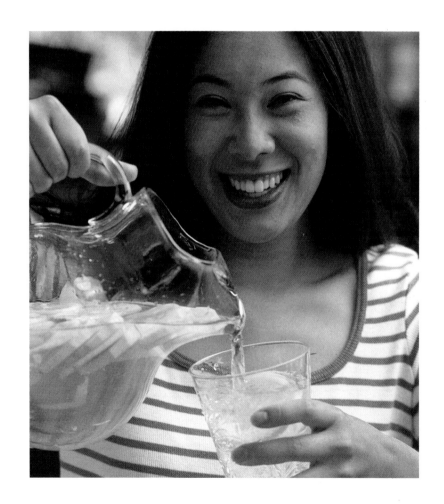

toners

Toners cleanse and refresh your skin. They are generally astringent, meaning they work to tighten your pores. Use a toner as part of your daily routine, applying it to your just-washed face to remove the last traces of your cleanser or scrub. You can also sweep a toner over your face as a mid-day freshener.

Most of the recipes on these pages make enough toner for many applications. Your homemade toners will last for a week in the refrigerator. Throw them out sooner if they start to look or smell funny.

Start looking for small, pretty bottles to store your toner in. You can always find small plastic bottles at a beauty supply store. Pour some toner into a pretty bottle, tie a ribbon around it and give it to a friend with instructions for using it.

Applying a toner

- Buy 100% cotton cosmetic pads to apply your toner. The fibers in regular facial tissue are scratchy and too harsh for your face.

- Pour enough toner onto the pad to dampen it almost completely.

- Sweep the toner-soaked cotton pad over your face, avoiding your eye area as always. If you do get toner in your eyes, rinse them immediately with water.

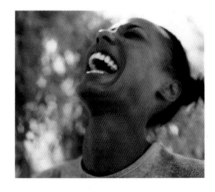

Fresh cucumber toner

One of the easiest toners ever. Cucumber juice is cool and soothing. Save the leftover cucumber in the fridge to use in another recipe or to make the spa water on page 25.

1 cucumber slice

Cut the cucumber slice into thirds.

Sweep the cucumber over your face and neck.

Splash your face with cool water, then pat dry.

Witch hazel is a wonderful natural astringent that is used in most of these recipes. Used undiluted it's an excellent toner, much gentler than pure alcohol. It's often mixed with other ingredients, which add their own toning qualities. You can buy witch hazel in most drugstores, usually in the same section where you'd find rubbing alcohol. If you don't find it, just ask. It's probably there somewhere.

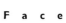

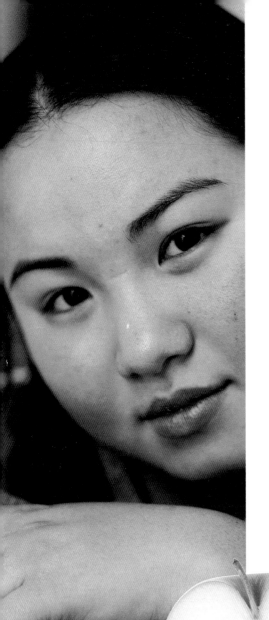

Citrus toner

Lemons and limes have natural antiseptic and astringent qualities. This toner works well on normal to oily skin.

juice from 1 lemon or lime
2 Tbsp witch hazel

Pour the ingredients into a bottle, cap it tightly, then shake to mix completely.

Apply as directed on page 26.

Apple toner

This gentle toner is a good choice if you have sensitive or fair skin.

¼ cup unsweetened apple juice
3 Tbsp witch hazel

Pour the ingredients into a bottle, cap it tightly, then shake to mix completely.

Apply as usual.

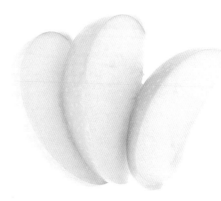

Minty toner

Peppermint is a naturally antiseptic tonic.

½ cup witch hazel
6–8 drops peppermint essential oil

Pour the ingredients into a bottle, cap it tightly, then shake to mix completely.

Apply as usual.

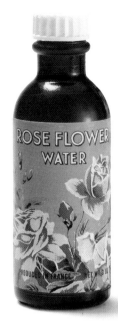

You may have to work a bit to find rosewater, but it's well worth the effort. You can often find it in drugstores, though you'll probably have better luck in natural food stores. Some cultures cook with rosewater, so if you have a grocery store with a good selection of international foods, try looking for it there. Be sure to buy the real thing. Imitation rosewater just isn't the same.

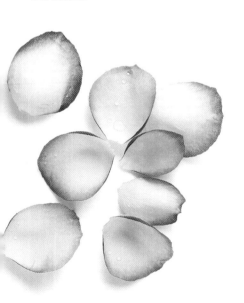

Rosewater toner

This is a wonderful, aromatic toner. The rosewater softens and soothes your skin.

Makes 4 ½ ounces.

¼ cup rosewater
3 Tbsp witch hazel

Pour the ingredients into a bottle, cap it tightly, then shake to mix completely.

Apply as directed on page 26.

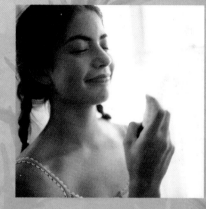

For a cool refresher, pour some of your favorite toner into a small spray bottle and store it in the fridge. Spritz the toner onto your face whenever you want a pick-me-up. On a hot day, nothing feels better.

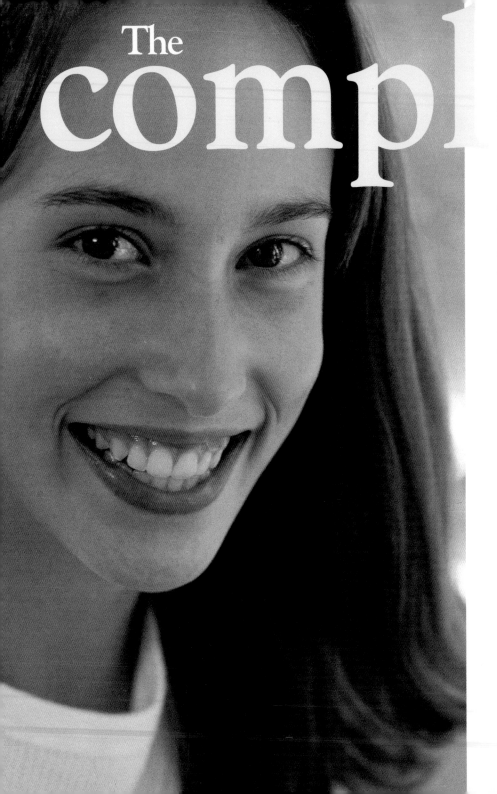

The complete

With the recipes in this chapter, you have everything you need to give a complete facial. You can give yourself a facial, but it's even better to trade facials with a friend. If you give yourself a facial, try doing it in the tub. In this case you don't need to plan a steam, as the warm bath water steams your face throughout your bath.

Getting ready

Choose a nice quiet room, where you have a place to lie down. A bed, a couch, or even the floor will work fine. Be sure to spread a clean towel over a pillow to protect from messy drips. Play some soothing music and keep the lights low if you can.

Find two clean washcloths. Get one wet with cold water, squeeze it out and place it in a bowl or plastic bag in the refrigerator to chill. Set the other washcloth aside for now. You'll probably want to have an extra towel around as well.

facial

Choose a recipe from each section

- scrub
- steam
- mask
- eye soother
- toner

Prepare each recipe before beginning the facial.

Fill a large bowl or pot with warm tap water and have this within reach as you give the facial.

Have your friend pull her hair back (the headband works well for this). Make sure her face is rinsed clean of any makeup. When that's done, she's ready to lie down and receive her facial.

The facial

- Dip the dry washcloth into the pot of warm water, then squeeze it out. Open the washcloth up and lay it across your friend's face for a moment to prepare her skin for the facial. Remove the washcloth before it cools.

- While her skin is still damp, apply the scrub, massaging it in circular motions all over her face. Use the warm washcloth to completely remove the scrub once you're finished.

- Next, have your friend sit up and steam her face for 10 minutes. Use this time to refresh the warm water in your bowl and to rinse out the washcloth. When she's finished with the steam, gently

pat her face dry with a clean towel, then have her lie back again to receive her mask.

- Apply the mask as directed. Place an eye soother over her eyes, and cover it with the washcloth from the fridge, folded into a band so it just covers her eyes. If you aren't using an eye soother, you can just lay the cool washcloth over her eyes.

- While the mask is working, give her a foot massage (page 49).

- When the mask is complete, remove the eye soothers, and use the washcloth and warm water to gently wipe her face clean of the mask.

- Finish by running a toner across her face with a cotton pad.

HAN &

SOAKS & HAND MASKS & MANICURE & FOOT SOAKS & EXFOLIANTS

DS FEET

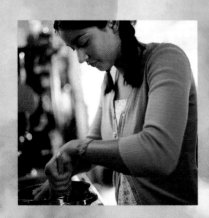

& MASSAGE & PEDICURE

A weekly manicure is a good way to keep your hands and nails looking their best. A basic manicure is as simple as cleaning and filing your nails and conditioning your cuticles.

Basic hand care

Filing

Always file your nails when they're dry. They'll be strongest if you file them into a blunt, squarish shape. File in one direction with light strokes. Never saw back and forth as this can cause your nails to split.

First file the ends straight across, always filing in the same direction...

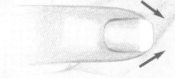

...then gently round the corners, filing from the outside towards the center of your nails.

Your hands will look best if your nails are all about the same length.

Cleaning

Use your nail brush to gently scrub your nails clean. Hold the brush at a 45-degree angle, and be careful not to push below the natural line of your nail. Scrub with baking soda and warm water to whiten your nails.

Cuticle care

Your cuticles create a seal between your nail and your finger. This seal keeps your nails healthy and strong. For this reason, don't cut into your cuticles. If you'd like to push them back, massage a little olive oil into them, gently pushing them back with your thumb as you do. Never use anything sharp to push your cuticles back.

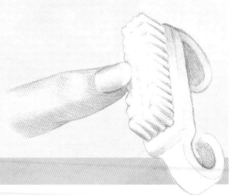

Moisturizing

Water is actually one of the most drying elements your hands come in contact with. Ideally, you should moisturize your hands every time you wash them. If this isn't doable, aim for at least twice a day.

soaks

The recipes on this page can be used alone or as part of a complete manicure.

Lemon soak

Lemon juice whitens your nails. Its antiseptic qualities help keep your nails healthy and strong.

*about 1 cup warm tap water
juice from ½ lemon
2–3 drops lavender essential oil
(optional but nice)*

Combine all the ingredients in a small bowl. Dip your nail brush into the solution to scrub your nails clean. Rinse your hands in warm tap water, then soak them in the leftover solution for 3–5 minutes per hand. Gently pat your hands dry.

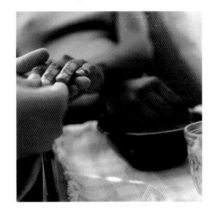

Buttermilk soak

Buttermilk whitens your nails and leaves your skin feeling soft and hydrated. This soak is especially nice if you warm the buttermilk just a little bit before soaking in it.

1 cup buttermilk, room temperature

Pour the buttermilk into a small bowl and soak your fingertips in it for about 5 minutes.

Intensive moisturizing soak

This mediterranean hand soak will soften your cuticles and moisturize your hands.

¼–⅓ cup olive oil

Pour some olive oil into a small bowl and soak each hand in it for at least one minute. Gently pat your hands dry with a tissue. If any oil remains rub it into your hands thoroughly.

YOUR NAILS GROW ABOUT ⅛ INCH A MONTH

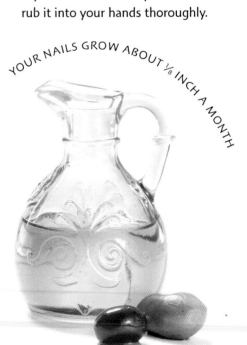

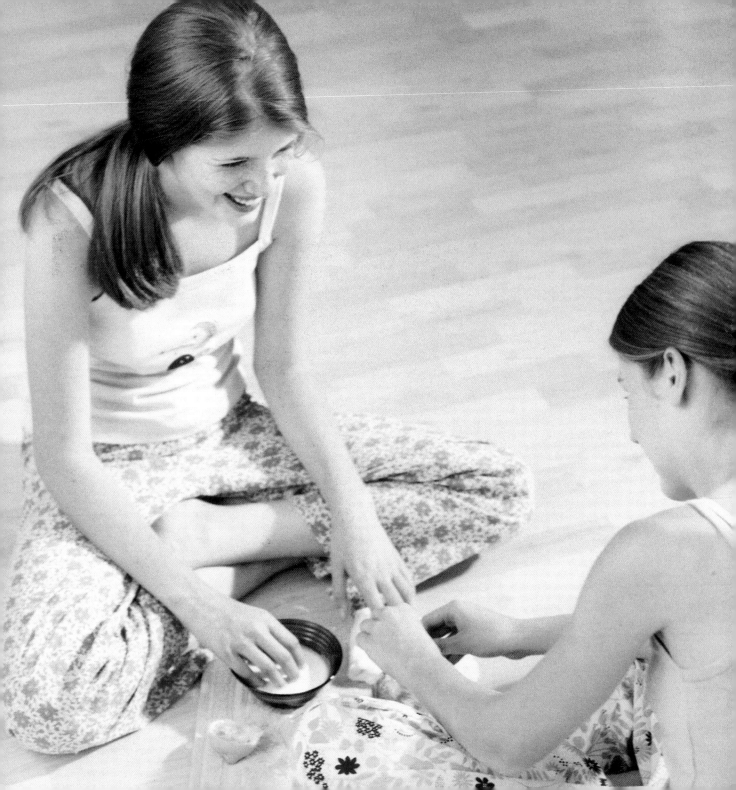

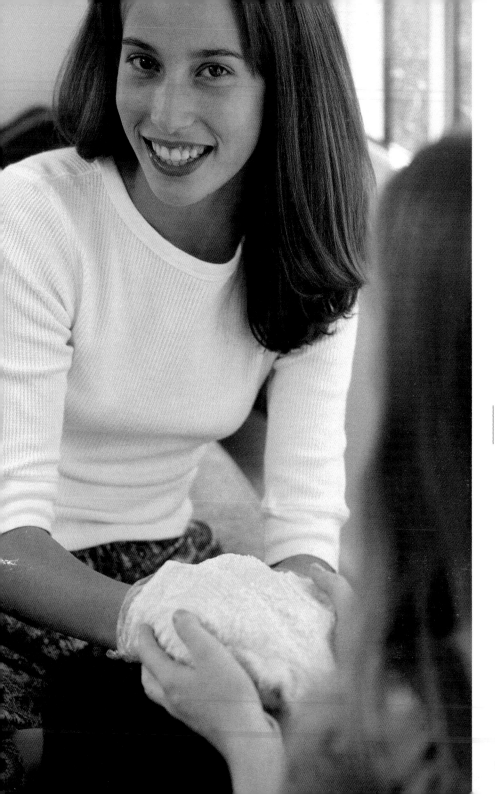

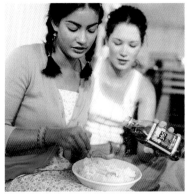

Mashed potato hand mask

*Potatoes and olive oil combine to make a
rich, moisturizing hand mask.*

2 potatoes
3 Tbsp olive oil

Cut the potatoes into quarters and
boil until soft. Drain them, then let
them sit until they're cool enough
to touch.

Mash the potatoes together with the
olive oil in a large bowl.

To use, dig your hands into the potatoes and work them all over your
hands, squeezing them between your
fingers. After about 5 minutes, rinse
your hands off in warm water and
gently pat dry. Throw the potatoes
away. Don't be tempted to eat them.

masks

Peaches and cream hand mask

Substitute a small handful of dried peaches or apricots if fresh fruit isn't available.

½ fresh peach
¼ cup plain yogurt, room
   temperature
1 Tbsp honey

Blend everything together, slather on your hands and let it sit for about 5 minutes before rinsing off.

Milk and honey hand mask

This mask softens and tones your hands and nails.

2 Tbsp whole yogurt or cream
1 Tbsp honey
1 Tbsp ground almonds
1 tsp rosewater (optional)

Rub the mask all over your hands to exfoliate, then let it sit for about 5 minutes before rinsing off.

Exfoliating hand mask

½ avocado
1 Tbsp cream, milk or yogurt
1 Tbsp cornmeal

Mash all the ingredients together in a small bowl. Rub the mask all over your hands to exfoliate. Then put each hand in a plastic bag and let them sit for about 5 minutes before rinsing off.

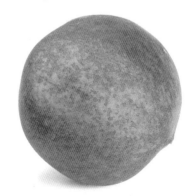

Warm hand mask

Adding heat to any hand mask makes it even more luxurious, and intensifies the moisturizing effects of the masks. This is easier to do if you have someone to help you. Prepare the mask of your choice, then gather two plastic bags and a hand towel. Run the hand towel under warm tap water, then squeeze it out. Apply the mask to your hands, working quickly so the towel doesn't cool. Tuck your mask-slathered hands into the plastic bags and wrap the warm towel around them. Let the mask sit for about 5 minutes or until the towel cools.

If you want to give yourself or a friend a complete manicure, this is what you do.

First, prepare all the recipes you plan on using. Spread a clean hand towel out on a table and gather everything you'll need. An extra towel, your file, a bowl for soaking, your nail brush and buffer. Work through the treatments in this order.

- file
- clean
- soak
- condition cuticles
- rub and/or mask
- buff

Healthy, clean, neatly shaped nails are beautiful just as they are. If you like to wear nail polish, know that both the polish and the remover can be pretty hard on your nails, drying and even discoloring them.

If you do paint your nails, give them an occasional rest by letting them go unpolished every couple of weeks. Rub a little tea tree oil (an essential oil) into your nails after using polish remover. Wipe yellowed nails with a little lemon juice or white cider vinegar. Be sure to moisturize them after doing this.

Buffing

Buffing is the last step in a natural manicure and is a healthy alternative to nail polish. The buffer smoothes and polishes your nails, leaving them naturally shiny.

Your buffer has three different sections: White smoothes, blue polishes and green shines. Start by running the white section lightly across each nail to reduce ridges and rough spots. Work in one direction. If your nails are especially thin, skip this step.

Now switch to the blue part of the buffer. Using the same light strokes, gently polish your nails.

Next, use the green side to buff your nails until they are smooth and glossy.

Finish by rubbing a drop of olive oil into each nail.

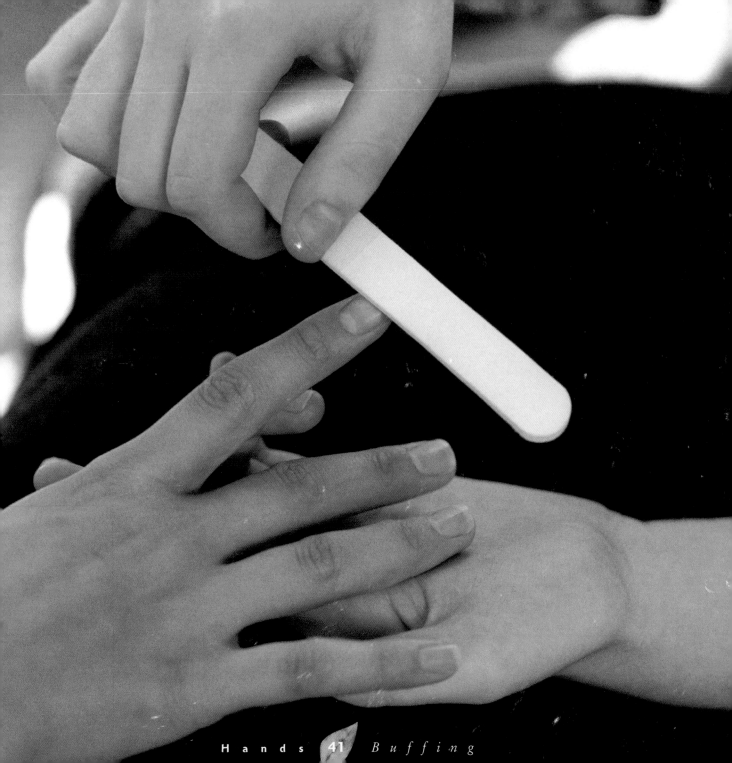

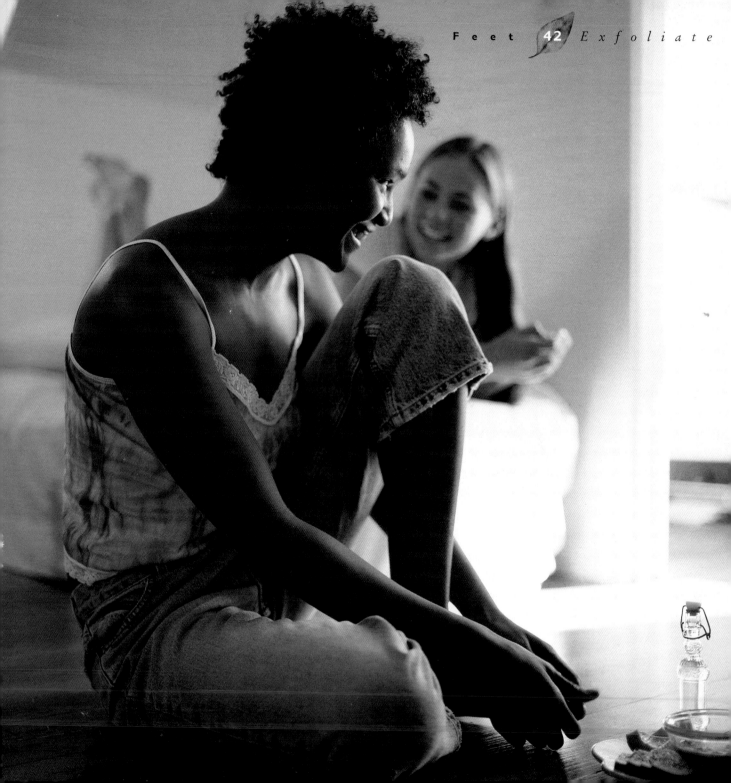

Your feet deserve more attention than they're getting now. It's just a fact. They work hard for you every day and deserve to be pampered now and then. Give yourself a weekly pedicure (page 49) or simply choose one of the treatments from this section for a quick foot reviver. As always, you can give yourself a pedicure, though it's nicer to trade with a friend.

The daily care of your feet is not much different from what you do for the rest of your body. Take a moment in the shower to wash your feet thoroughly.

Afterwards, dry them completely, being sure to get between each toe. Dust them with a little powder or cornstarch afterwards to be sure they're really dry.

One more thought to add to the list of things you already know, but probably need to hear again: Comfortable shoes are just the best. Give up those shoes that look good but feel bad. Your feet will thank you.

Trimming

It's best to keep your toenails short. Use nail scissors or clippers to cut them straight across, leaving just a narrow edge of white nail showing.

Cleaning

Use your nail brush to clean your toenails just like you did your fingernails.

Smoothing

Rub your pumice stone over rough spots on your feet to remove hard, dead skin. Always do this while your feet are damp (just after a soak or while you're in the tub).

Don't expect to remove all the dead skin the first time you do this. This treatment works best if repeated regularly over time.

soaks

Soaks are a wonderful way to cleanse and soothe tired feet. Even if you think your feet aren't tired, they probably are. Try one of these soaks and your feet will thank you.

Soak

- You'll need a basin big enough to hold your feet and deep enough to fill to about ankle height. Find a comfortable place to sit and spread a towel out where the basin will go. Have an extra towel on hand to dry your feet after the soak.

- Soak your clean feet for about 5-10 minutes, then rinse and dry completely.

Pineapple soak

Pineapple contains an enzyme which breaks down dead skin cells. This soak is especially effective when followed with a smoothing and exfoliating treatment.

warm tap water
2 cups pineapple juice

Pour the juice into the basin then add enough warm water to fill the basin about halfway. Soak your feet for 5-10 minutes. Follow with a pumice smoothing treatment or a sugar rub for best effect.

Minty foot soak

This is a refreshing foot soak, perfect as part of a full pedicure or all on its own.

warm tap water
3 herbal mint tea bags

Place the tea bags in the basin, then fill it about halfway with warm water. Ideally the water should come up to your ankles. Soak your feet in the warm water for 5-10 minutes.

Lavender salt soak

Epsom salts soothe aching, tired feet and reduce swelling. Buy Epsom salts at a drugstore, and be sure to read the manufacturer's label.

¼ cup Epsom salts
warm tap water
5-10 drops of lavender essential oil (or the essential oil of your choice)

Pour the salt into the basin, then add enough warm water to fill about halfway. Add the essential oil and soak your feet for 5-10 minutes.

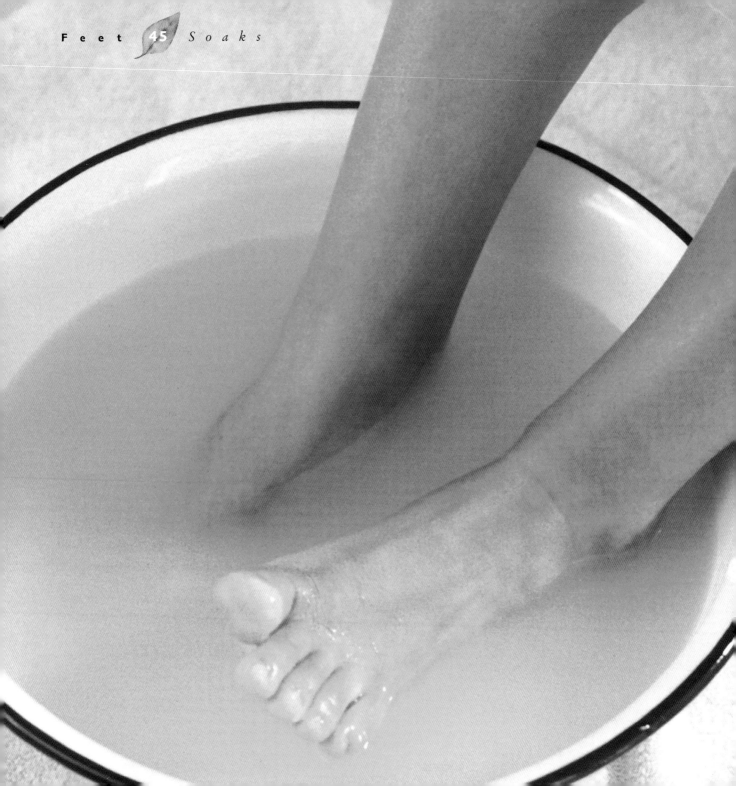

Use one of these exfoliating scrubs to smooth and soften your feet.

- Choose and prepare a recipe.

- Rub the mixture briskly all over your feet and up to your ankles. This is messy so do it over the tub or a towel.

- Rinse your feet in warm water then dry completely.

Sugar scrub

This recipe is a great way to soften your feet. The sugar and lemon exfoliate and revitalize your skin while the oil moisturizes. Halve the recipe if you want to use it on your hands as part of a manicure.

½ cup granulated sugar
1 Tbsp oil (almond, canola, avocado or olive oil)
juice from ½ lemon

Combine the ingredients in a medium-sized bowl.

Get your feet slightly wet, then apply the scrub as directed in the basic instructions.

Banana moisturizing exfoliant

This is a rich moisturizing exfoliator.

1 ripe banana, mashed
¼ cup ground almonds (in a pinch you can substitute cornmeal)
2 Tbsp whole oats

Combine all the ingredients in a bowl then rub briskly all over your feet, paying special attention to rough spots. If you have time, put your banana-coated feet in a plastic bag and wrap in a warm damp towel for about 5 minutes to intensify this treatment's moisturizing effects. Rinse and dry your feet.

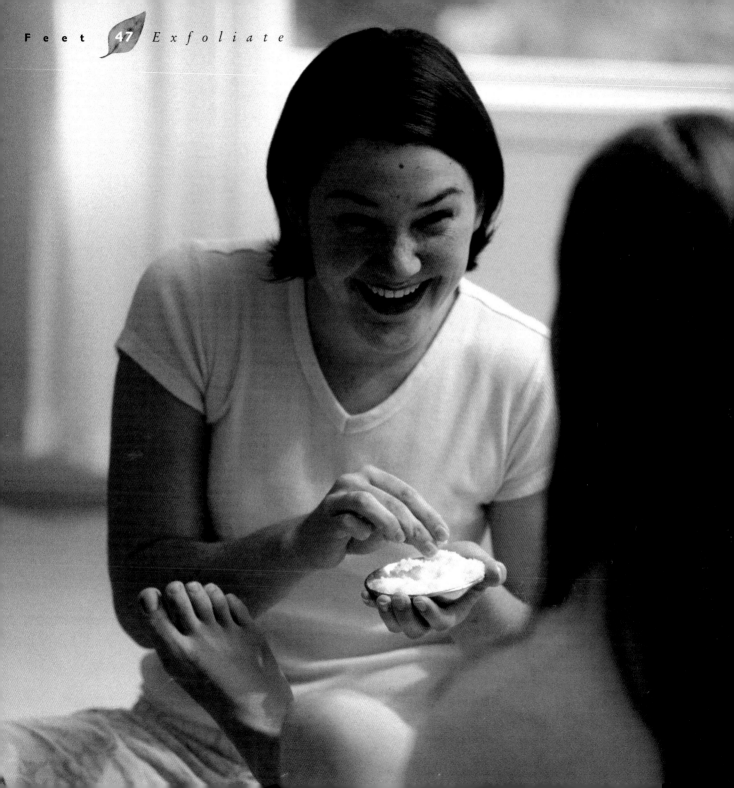

massage

Overnight moisturizer

**If your feet are especially dry, try
slathering them with massage oil or
simple olive oil before you go to bed.
Put on a pair of old cotton socks to
protect your sheets and let the
treatment work while you sleep.**

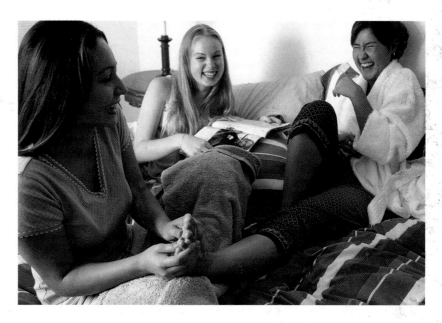

Finish your pedicure with a final moisturizing massage. While it's always more fun to have someone else give you a foot massage, you can easily massage your own feet.

Massage oil

Use a light, unscented oil like canola, safflower, or apricot kernel oil. Pour some into a small bottle and add a few drops of your favorite essential oil if you'd like. You can also use your favorite lotion or cream.

The perfect pedicure
- soak
- trim & clean nails
- smooth
- exfoliate
- massage & moisturize

Massage

Pour a few drops of oil into the palm of your hand and rub your hands together to warm them and coat them with oil. You may need to apply more oil during the massage. Rub your hands briskly all over your foot to increase the circulation.

Hold your foot in one hand and rotate it several times in both directions to loosen your ankle.

Rub your thumbs over the arch of your foot, starting just above your heel and working up to just below the ball of your foot.

Press your thumbs deeply all over the ball of your foot up to the base of your toes.

Massage each toe individually, starting at the base of the toe and massaging firmly as you gently pull on the toe and work your way out to the tip.

Run your thumb firmly along the sides of the foot and around your ankle bone.

Still awake? Move on to the other foot.

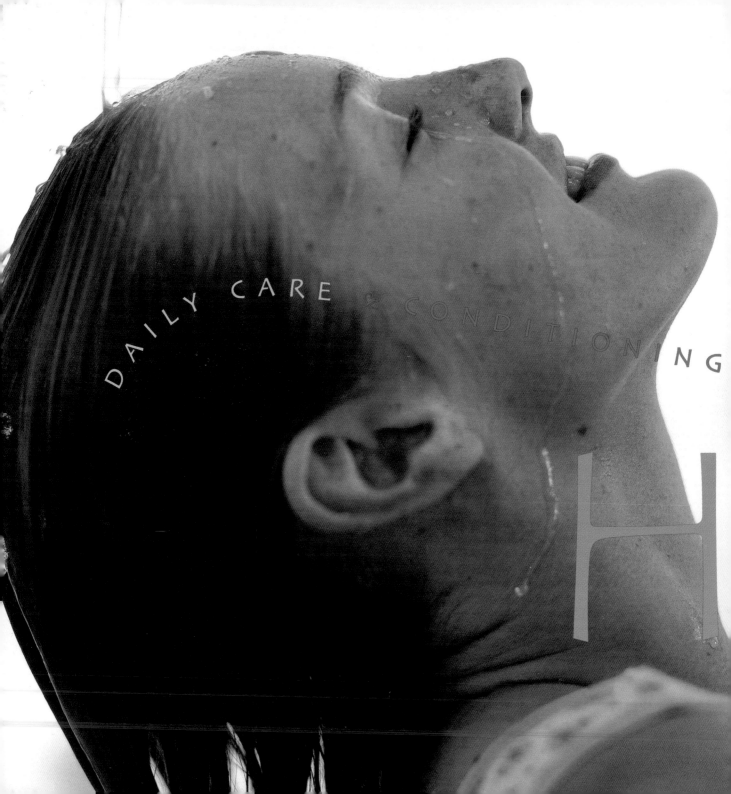

DAILY CARE & CONDITIONING

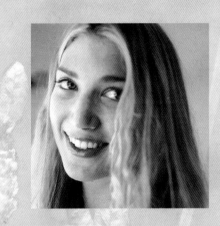

MASKS & RINSES

AIR

The less you do to your hair, the healthier it will be. Don't over-wash it, limit your use of gels and sprays and — most important — avoid heat. In an ideal world, you would never subject your hair to the effects of blow dryers, hot curlers or curling irons.

The reality is that you probably do some or all of these things to your hair. That's OK. You can still improve the health of your hair with the natural hair treatments in this section. Start with these basics of hair care.

It's generally enough to wash your hair every other day. The only exception is for swimmers, who should wash with a gentle shampoo every time they climb out of the pool. If you exercise every day, try washing your hair with shampoo one day and simply rinsing and conditioning the next. Washing your hair too often can overstimulate your scalp, causing it to produce more oil. Just what you don't want.

Whenever possible, let your hair air dry.

Keep your ends healthy by trimming them about every 6 weeks.

Washing your hair
- Before shampooing, brush or comb your hair to untangle it.
- Get your hair thoroughly wet.
- Pour a small amount of shampoo into the palm of your hand. A dollop the size of a nickel is about right. Use a little more if your hair is extra long, less if it's really short.
- Rub your hands together to distribute the shampoo then massage it into your scalp. Use your fingertips to really massage your whole scalp. It'll feel great.
- Next, work the shampoo gently down to the ends of your hair. Don't scrub your hair or bunch it up. Treat it gently. The ends don't need much shampooing.
- Rinse your hair thoroughly to remove all the shampoo.
- Follow with a detangling conditioner if you like.
- After gently toweling your hair dry, comb it out with a wide-toothed comb.

care

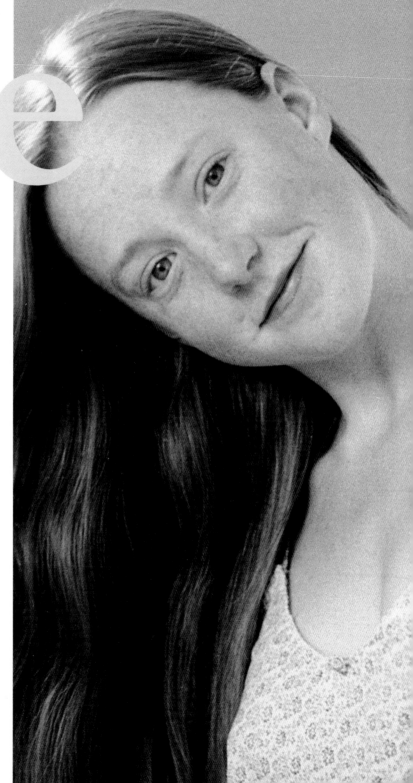

Super-clean shampoo

Products like gel and hair spray — even some shampoos and conditioners — leave a residue behind that can make your hair look dull. Try adding a teaspoon of baking soda to your shampoo once a week to remove this build-up and leave your hair clean and shiny.

Natural setting spritzer

Lemon juice is a natural replacement for setting gel or hair spray. Simply pour some fresh lemon juice into a small spray bottle and spritz it onto your hair before curling. You can also spray it on your already-styled hair to hold it lightly in place. As always, be careful not to get lemon juice in your eyes. Lemon juice lasts about a week in the refrigerator.

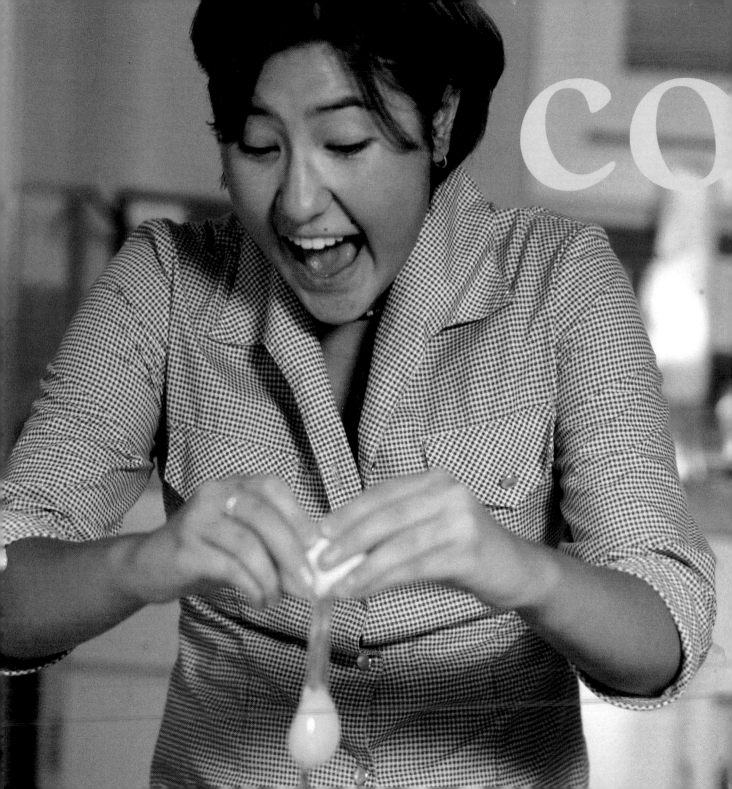

CO

These intensive conditioning hair masks can be used as often as once a week to condition and revitalize your hair. They're especially good to add to your routine if you regularly blow-dry your hair.

Applying a conditioning mask

- Always apply your hair mask to wet hair before shampooing.
- Work the mask over your scalp and down to the ends of your hair. Cover your hair with a shower cap and let the mask work for 10–15 minutes.
- To intensify the treatment, wrap a warm, just-out-of-the-dryer towel around your head turban-style. A warm, damp towel also works.
- Rinse your hair in warm water, then shampoo it thoroughly.

Banana deep conditioner

This tropical treatment conditions your hair and scalp.

1 ripe banana
1 egg yolk
1 Tbsp honey

Mash everything together in a bowl until smooth. You can use a blender to do this if you'd like. Follow the directions for applying a hair mask. Always keep raw eggs away from cuts and scrapes.

Avocado ginger hair mask

The ginger stimulates your scalp while the avocado moisturizes. Sesame oil is best, but it's OK to substitute another oil if you need to.

1 avocado
1 tsp powdered ginger
1 tsp sesame oil

Mash everything together to make a smooth puree. Apply as usual, then wash your hair thoroughly.

Lavender oil treatment

Lavender and olive oil strengthen your hair and prevent split ends.

1/4 cup olive oil
6 drops lavender essential oil

Combine the oils in a plastic container. Apply to your hair as always, then shampoo your hair thoroughly.

Egg conditioning mask

This rich mask leaves your hair shiny and soft. Be sure to rinse your hair with warm (not hot) water. Otherwise you'll find yourself with a head full of scrambled eggs. Always keep raw egg away from broken skin.

1 egg
1 tsp lemon juice

Whisk the egg until frothy. Stir in the lemon juice, then apply as you would any hair mask. Rinse your hair in warm water then shampoo thoroughly.

rinse

Hair rinses provide a good finishing touch to your hair care routine. It's best to give yourself a rinse in the tub or shower, pouring the rinse over your hair at the scalp and letting it run all the way down to the ends of your hair. These recipes make enough for one rinse.

Chamomile rinse

This rinse brings out the highlights in blond and red hair. Use it as a final rinse and it will leave your hair shiny and softly scented.

2 cups water
2 chamomile tea bags

Bring the water to a boil. Add the tea bags, cover the pot and let the rinse cool completely. Remove the tea bags. Pour the rinse over your hair after shampooing and conditioning. Leave it in as a final rinse.

Rosemary rinse

This rinse adds luster to dark hair.

1 cup water
3 Tbsp dried rosemary or (even better) a couple sprigs fresh rosemary
1 cup cider vinegar

Place the water and rosemary in a small pot and bring to a boil. Remove from heat and add the vinegar. Let the rinse sit until it's completely cool. Strain the rosemary out and discard. Pour the rinse over your hair after shampooing and conditioning. Be careful not to get it in your eyes. After about 5 minutes rinse your hair thoroughly in warm water.

Lemon lightening rinse

Lemon rinses your hair clean and lightens it as well.

juice from one lemon
2 cups warm water

Combine the water and lemon juice. Pour over your hair after shampooing and conditioning as a final rinse. Avoid getting this rinse in your eyes. It will sting.

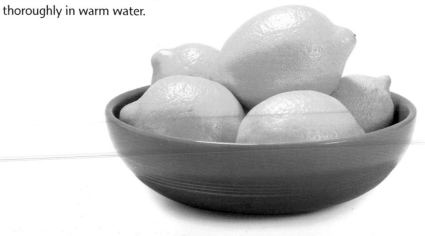

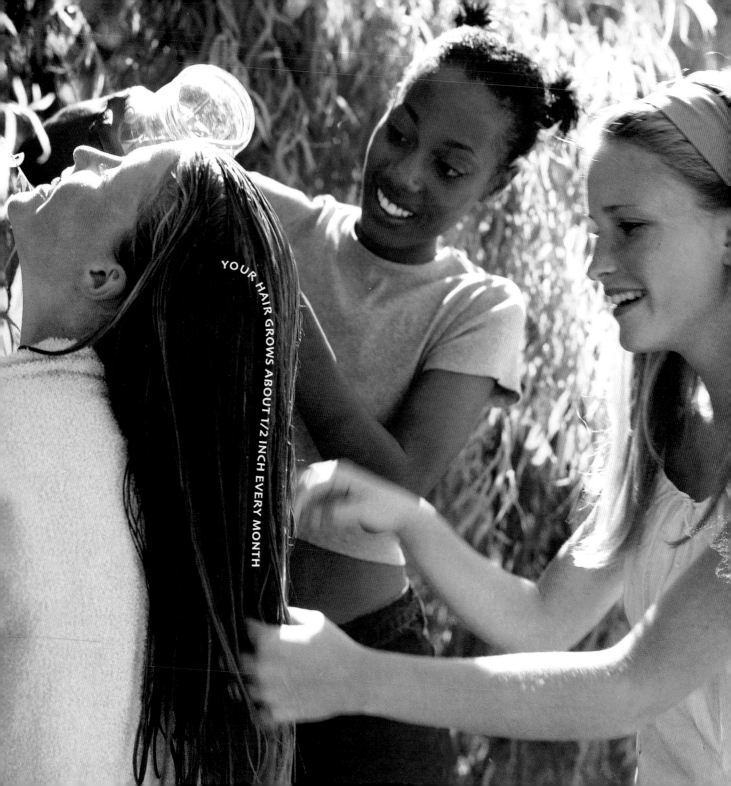

YOUR HAIR GROWS ABOUT 1/2 INCH EVERY MONTH

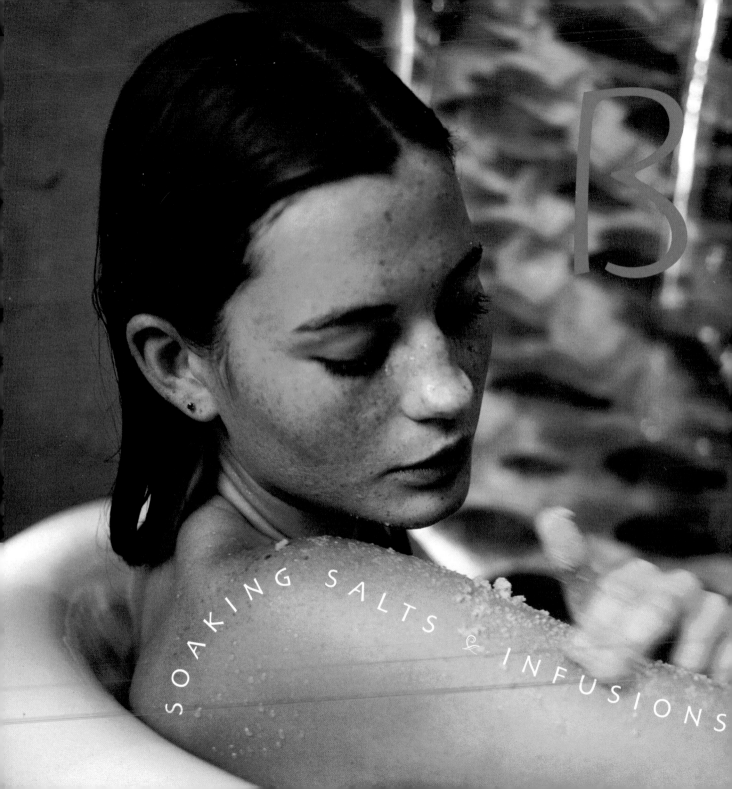

3

SOAKING SALTS & INFUSIONS

ATH

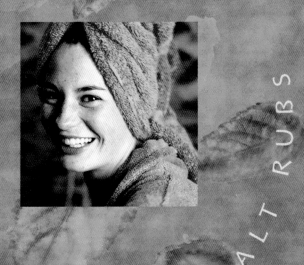

BATH FIZZES & SALT RUBS

bath

Bath salts have been used for years as a soothing therapy for skin. We use Epsom salts, which are especially good for relieving achy muscles and joints. You'll find them at your local drugstore. Just ask. They have them somewhere. Always read the label of commercial products carefully and store as directed. Coarse sea salt (available at the grocery store) also works.

You can store your bath salts indefinitely in an airtight container, though their scent will fade over time.

Basic bath salt

2 cups Epsom salts
6–7 drops essential oil
(Choose one scent, or blend a couple.)

Pour the salt into a large jar, add the essential oil and put a lid on the jar. Shake the salt to distribute the scent. It's nice, but not essential, to let the bath salts sit overnight before using them, so the oil really seeps into the salt.

Add about 1/2 cup to your tub once it's filled with water. Swish it around a little so that it dissolves before you get in. Climb in and relax.

Fresh milk bath

Milk baths soften your skin.

1 qt whole milk
5–6 drops essential oil

Add the oil to the milk and give it all a little shake. Pour the milk into the tub while it's filling.

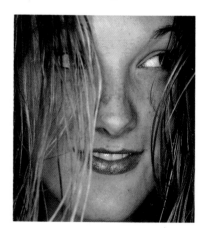

MOISTURIZE YOUR SKIN AFTER USING BATH SALTS

salts

Mineral milk bath

This bath is especially good if your skin is itchy or irritated. But don't just save it for these situations. It's also a very gentle everyday bath.

1½ cup dried milk (powdered, non-instant brands are best)
½ cup baking soda
6–10 drops of essential oil

Pour the milk and baking soda into a large jar, add the essentail oil and cover tightly. Shake well to mix it all up. Store in an airtight container. Add about 1 cup to your bath water.

Ginger honey bath

This bath is especially soothing when you're feeling achy. Don't be surprised if it makes your skin tingle a little. If you find it uncomfortable, simply rinse off.

2 Tbsp ground ginger
¼ cup honey

Add the ginger and honey to the tub while it's filling. Pour it right under the flow of water, then swish it around to mix it all up.

Coloring your bath salts

If you want to color your bath salts, simply add a few drops of food coloring to the salt, put it in a jar with a lid, and shake until the salt is pretty evenly colored. Try layering two different colors of salt in one bottle. A jar of bath salts, tied with a ribbon, makes a great gift.

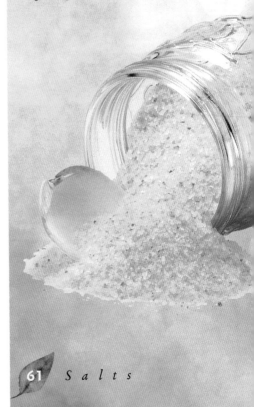

SPRINKLE SWEET-SMELLING ROSE PETALS INTO YOUR BATH FOR A SPECIAL TREAT

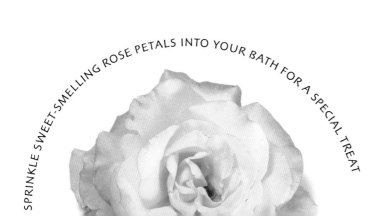

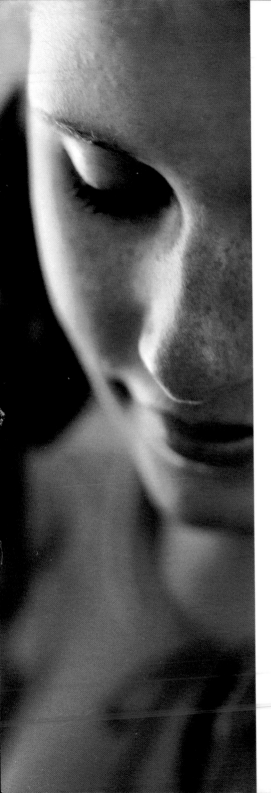

Tub infusions turn every bath into an aromatherapy treatment.

Using an infusion

- Mix your infusion.

- Find the little muslin tea bag that came with this book. This is your tub tea bag and you won't want to lose it.

- Fill the bag about 3/4 full with the infusion of your choice.

- Tie the bag closed, then drop it in the tub while it fills with hot water.

- Once in the tub, you can squeeze the bag to help release the scent.

- After your bath, throw away the contents of the bag, turn the bag inside out and rinse it well. Hang it up to dry until you're ready to use it again.

Herbal infusion

You can use one herb, or combine several to make your personal blend. Fresh herbs are always best, but dried herbs also work fine.

handful rosemary and/or sage

Put the herbs in your bag and follow the directions for using an infusion.

Lemon mint infusion

This is an especially refreshing summer infusion.

½ lemon, sliced
a handful fresh or dried mint

Put the mint and lemon in your tea bag and follow the directions for using an infusion.

Lavender oat infusion

This recipe makes enough for several infusions. Store the leftovers in a cool dry place.

After the bag has soaked in the tub for a few minutes, wipe it over your skin like a washcloth to get the full softening benefits of the oats. Look for dried lavender flowers in natural food stores or bath shops. If you can't find them, just add a few drops of lavender essential oil.

1 cup uncooked oatmeal
1 cup dried lavender blossoms

Combine the two ingredients and store in an airtight jar until you're ready to use. Then scoop some of the mixture into your bag and follow the basic instructions for an infusion.

Single-use lavender oat infusions

Make individual lavender oat infusions to give as gifts. Simply buy paper coffee filters for an automatic coffee maker (chances are good you already have some in the house). Put a handful of infusion into the filter and tie it closed with a ribbon. Attach instructions to add a bag to the bath while it's filling. Afterwards, the infusion can be thrown away.

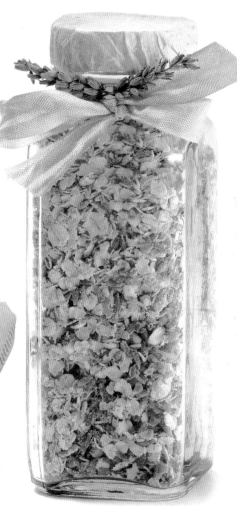

Lavender
Oat Infusion
- Drop bag into tub.
- Climb in.
- Relax.

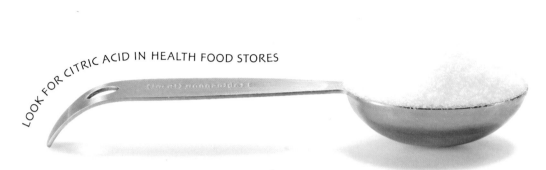

LOOK FOR CITRIC ACID IN HEALTH FOOD STORES

This is a fun way to scent and soften your bath water. You'll need to buy some citric acid for this recipe. It might take a little work to find it, but these fizzes are well worth the effort. Call around to natural food stores in your area. If they don't have it in stock, they'll probably order it for you.

Bath fizz

- 1 cup baking soda
- 3 Tbsp citric acid
- 3 Tbsp corn starch
- 3 Tbsp plus 1 tsp light oil (canola, apricot kernel, almond)
- 6 drops essential oil
- a few drops food coloring (optional)

Pour all the dry ingredients into a bowl and combine well. Add the oils, then use your hands to mix everything really well. Press handfuls of the mixture firmly between the palms of your hands to make 5–6 rounds. The mixture will be crumbly. If it doesn't hold together, add a few more drops of oil.

Put on a plate in a cool dry place and let them sit for 2 days to harden. This takes a little patience but it's an important step.

After 2 days, you can wrap them individually in waxed paper or place them in an airtight jar and store in the fridge. It's best to use them within a few weeks. If they get too old the oil may turn bad (you'll know by the smell if this has happened).

TO USE A FIZZ: Fill your tub with water and climb in. Drop one or two fizzes in the tub, lie back and enjoy the effervescence.

WRAP YOUR FIZZES INDIVIDUALLY IN WAXED PAPER, THEN IN PRETTY PAPER TIED WITH A RIBBON. GIVE THEM AS GIFTS.

Bath Fizz

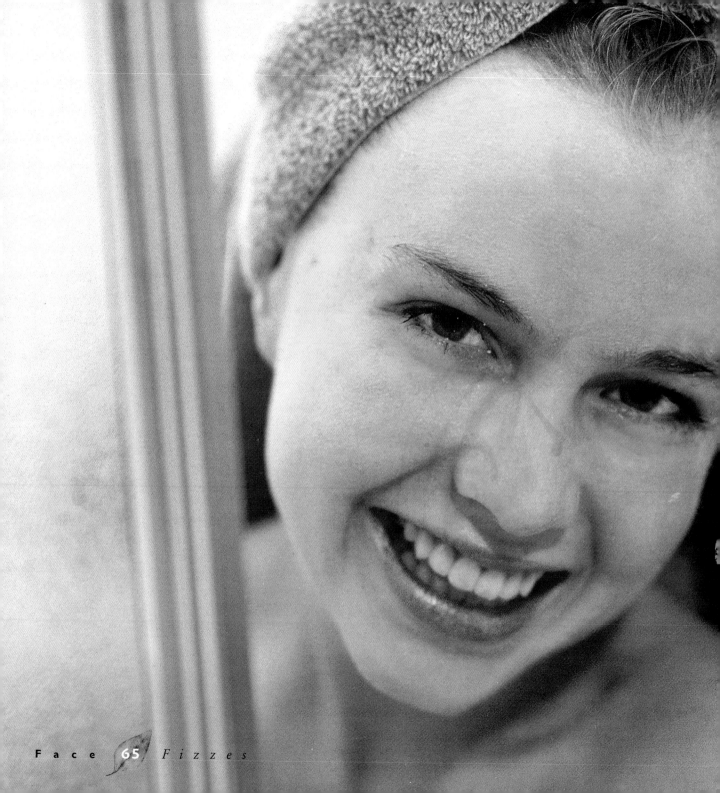

salt

If you've never given yourself a salt rub, you've been missing out. Big time. A good salt rub does it all: It energizes and invigorates your skin, it sloughs off dead cells and it leaves your skin moisturized and positively glowing. Using one of these rubs on your legs before shaving will give you a closer, smoother shave. Are you convinced yet?

Give yourself a salt rub in the tub. One word of caution: Salt rubs make the tub slippery. Be very careful when standing in a tub after a rub, and clean out the bath afterwards so no one else is surprised by a slippery tub.

Buy fine sea salt at the grocery store. It's easy to find.

You can use any of these recipes as part of a pedicure (after soaking).

Giving yourself a salt rub

- Put your already-made salt rub in a plastic cup or jar (never take glass into the tub). These recipes make enough for one or two rubs. Store leftovers in the fridge for up to a month.

- Soak in your bath for a moment so that your skin is completely wet.

- Rub small handfuls of the salt all over your body in brisk circular motions. Pay special attention to rough spots like elbows and heels. Avoid your face and any cuts or scratches. Rinse off.

- You won't need to moisturize after your bath. The salt rub will leave your skin soft and moisturized.

Aloe salt rub

This rub is a little lighter than the other rubs and takes advantage of aloe vera's skin-soothing qualities. Look for aloe vera gel in the suntan section of your drugstore or in natural food stores.

1 cup fine sea salt
1 Tbsp aloe vera gel
1 Tbsp light oil (canola, apricot kernel, almond)

Pour the salt into a medium-sized bowl and add the oils. Use your hands to mix the ingredients together well. Store in a covered plastic container until you're ready to use.

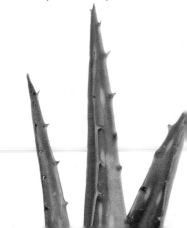

rubs

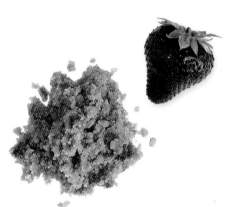

Peppermint salt rub

Peppermint is an energizing tonic for your skin.

1 cup fine sea salt
2 Tbsp light oil (canola, apricot kernel, almond)
5–6 drops peppermint essential oil (or experiment with different scents)

Put the salt in a medium-sized bowl and add the oils. Use your hands to mix the ingredients together well. Store in a covered plastic container until you're ready to use.

Strawberry salt rub

This is quite simply the best recipe in the book. Smells great, looks great, feels great. If strawberries aren't in season, use a couple of thawed frozen ones. Depending on the ripeness of the strawberries, the rub will be bright pink or light purple. Either color is fine. Raspberries also make a wonderful substitution.

1 cup fine sea salt
3 ripe strawberries
1 Tbsp light oil (canola, apricot kernel, almond)

Pour the salt into a medium-sized bowl and add the oil and strawberries. Mash everything together with a fork. Use your hands if necessary to really blend the strawberries in with the salt. Store in a covered plastic container until you're ready to use. This will keep in the fridge for a couple of weeks, but you'll want to use it faster than that! Yum.

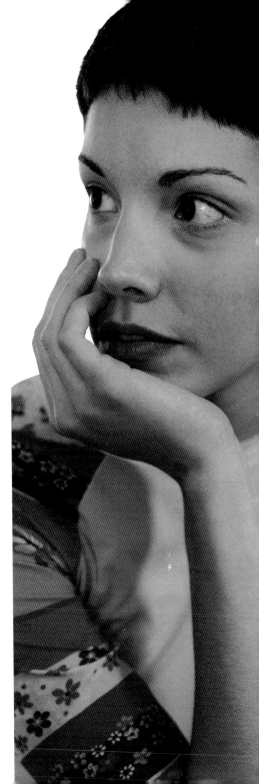

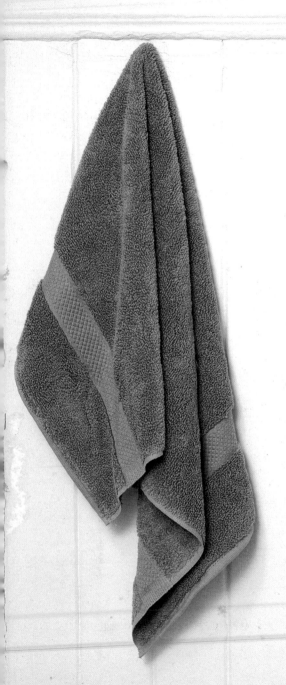

KLUTZ®

**455 Portage Avenue
Palo Alto, CA 94306
(650) 857-0888** KLUTZ.com

Design and Production
Jami Spittler, Jamison Design

Photography
Peter Fox
Thomas Heinser
Jock McDonald
Judy Swinks
Richard Reader

Illustrations
Don Bishop

Technical Illustrations
Sara Boore

Casting and Editorial Assistance
Corie Thompson

Models
Stacy Alo, Charlene Ayers, Danielle Bassett, Christina Belen, Jennifer Bellotti, Jessica Bellotti, Andrea Benetez, Jasmine Chan, Larkin Clark, Molly Anne Coogan, Kelly Curran, Sarah Espinoza, Jennifer Foster, Sydney Garrison, Katie Gutierrez, Carly Helsaple, Elva Kirtland, Michelle Mayberry, Chetna Mehta, Paulina Morales, Anais Morgan, Honee Nuriddin, Tandem Ogilvie, Elena Praskin, Johanna Rompf, Joel' Rutsky, Angela Salvidar, Allysa Taylor Scott, Shay, Dana Shew, Tiffany Simon, Katie Sticksel, Katy Svetlichny, Zoe Swenson-Graham, Erica Yarbrough.

Special thanks to all the brave testers in the Klutz office.